Whole Food Diet

Healthy Eating

By Cathy Wilson

Copyright © 2015

Income Disclaimer

This book contains business strategies, marketing methods and other business advice that, regardless of my own results and experience, may not produce the same results (or any results) for you. I make absolutely no guarantee, expressed or implied, that by following the advice below you will make any money or improve current profits, as there are several factors and variables that come into play regarding any given business.

Primarily, results will depend on the nature of the product or business model, the conditions of the marketplace, the experience of the individual, and situations and elements that are beyond your control.
As with any business endeavor, you assume all risk related to investment and money based on your own discretion and at your own potential expense.

Liability Disclaimer
By reading this book, you assume all risks associated with using the advice given below, with a full understanding that you, solely, are responsible for anything that may occur as a result of putting this information into action in any way, and regardless of your interpretation of the advice.
You further agree that our company cannot be held responsible in any way for the success or failure of your business as a result of the information presented in this book. It is your responsibility to conduct your own due diligence regarding the safe and successful operation of your business if you intend to apply any of our information in any way to your business operations.

Terms of Use

Whole Food Diet
Healthy Eating

By Cathy Wilson

Table of Contents

Introduction

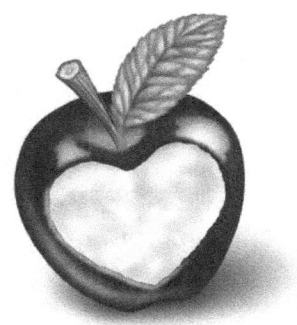

The Whole Food Diet will . . .
Enable more efficient BRAIN function
Deter body breakdown and build it strong
Support healthy WEIGHT
Relax your MIND and reduce STRESS naturally
Remind your TASTEBUDS that healthy eating is tasty
Are you going to keep allowing extrinsic societal pressures to dictate your health and wellness?

FACT - *Dr. OZ, WebMD*, and oodles of health professionals, recommend eating a diet of mainly **whole foods,** to attain optimal health long-term.

CIP - Cathy's Important Point - This **evolutionary science-based** eating plan **WILL** improve your health mentally, socially, physically, and environmentally.

My making the conscious decision to take back your good health by eating healthy whole food choices and exercising regularly, you WILL...

*Lose pesky fat FAST
*Build lean sexy muscle
*Improve your heart and lung function
*Build your body resistant to serious disease
*Lower your risk of cardiovascular disease and stroke
*Improve memory
*Extend life expectancy
*LIVE INDEPENDENT LONGER
*Disable annoying chronic pain
And so much more!

We live in a crazy fast paced world that leaves little room for *au natural*. The faster the better. This means modified foods too. You aren't conditioned to make time to prepare natural and wholesome food meals, because it's so much easier to scoot through the drive thru. Not make the time to grab some fresh fruit from a garden market.

Instead, you'll pop a few coins into the vending machine and down a pastry.
It doesn't take long for this scenario to manifest into habit, and the rest is history!

Poor eating habits and little or no regular exercise results in obesity. This triggers all sorts of serious health issues, including diabetes, stroke, and cardiovascular disease to start.

These preventable issues steal your quality of life and more. And for the most part are absolute. The super sad part is, most disease is preventable. If we take action as a society, focusing on prevention, we'll avoid lots of un-necessary deaths and broken hearts.

Choosing to get healthy by going back in time to exercising regularly, and making Whole Food Plant Based Diet choices for eating, will turn your world right-side-up.

You'll...
*Lose fat permanently
*Gain energy
*Become more productive
*Decrease mood swings
*Think with clarity
*Lower the risk of serious disease
*Release that "feel good" feeling
*Ease stress just knowing you're eating healthy

By implementing the Whole Food Diet into your everyday, along with a healthy interval training exercise, you **WILL** succeed in long-term weight loss, and overall great health and wellness.

My fantabulous introductory book is ready to get you started!

Whole Foods Explained

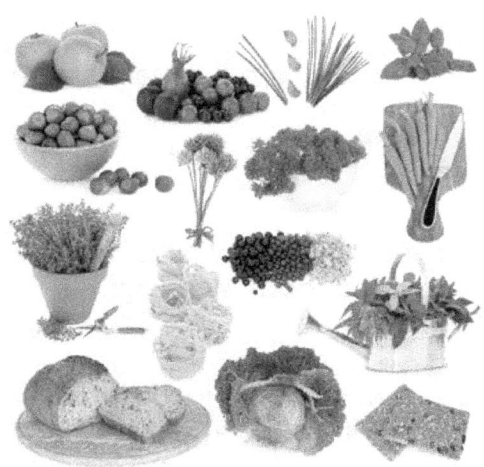

Whole foods are foods which are all-natural, unpro-
cessed and unrefined, as much as possible. Avoid
additives and preservatives, including added fat, salt and
carbohydrates.

Rewinding time, all foods used to be whole, including unpasteurized milk products. Experts agree, food
processing which involves the addition of numerous
chemicals and preservatives, negatively impacts your
health. Heart disease, high blood pressure, cancer,
stroke, and many other serious diseases are linked to
chemically- altered processed foods.

Rule of Thumb - *If the food isn't packaged and doesn't
come with an ingredient list, it's in a natural state with
nothing added. You've got the green light to eat up!*

Many people are confused whole foods are **always** organic.

Organic foods *are produced, manufactured and handled, following the USDA guide with regards to organic foods.*

Natural or Whole foods *are not mandated by this process.*

Beware organic food isn't always whole, and whole food isn't always organic.

Am I confusing you? Because I'm confusing myself! Just remember **whole foods** and **organic foods** should be your first choice!

VIP - Enzymes found in whole foods are critical in all chemical processes in your body, particularly when it comes to digesting food. If you add the heating of processed foods, chemicals and preservatives and other toxins to the mix, you're creating more volatile and destructive chemical reactions, taking away the health benefits of the foods you're consuming.

Scientific research shows these triggered unnatural chemical reactions have dangerous effects on your health. Even just cooking some foods can create negative chemical reactions.

For instance, heating carbohydrates, like in processed and packaged high-fat simple carbs, transforms carbohydrate molecules into carcinogens called acrylamide. A chemical used in plastics and dyes that causes cancer in animals.

We want convenience, and have conditioned ourselves to ignore healthy whole foods, and opt for the sugar laden, high-fat, unhealthy *fast* foods. All of which interfere with the smooth running of your intricate bodily systems, creating disease, illness, and eventually death.

This isn't something you can fix with a Band-Aid. If you want to gain control of your health, it's time to make the commitment to do it right. This means you've got to make the mental, physical, and emotional changes to make whole food eating your new *normal*.

To repeat the same actions and expect a different result is insane!
Is this going to take time? That's a big **YES**.

Are you going to need patience, perseverance, support, and expert knowledge (Cathy) to make it easier? That's affirmative.

By understanding what whole foods are, and how they benefit your health; mind, body and soul, you'll see making the switch to whole food eating really is a no-brainer. Don't try and be perfect.

Change is hard.
Take it one step at a time and set yourself up for success. Learn to implement manageable changes that'll stick for your lifetime. Seeing is believing for most of us. Slowly but surely by choosing whole food eating, you'll look and feel differently. This fuels your desire to make positive changes in your eating. That's just the way the cookie crumbles, or should I say, banana gets peeled! Whole foods used to be the only way people ate. They had no choice. Now we've oodles of choice, and it's up to you to pick wise-owl wisely. You can continue eating processed and unhealthy toxic foods that are *knowingly*

destroying your body and mind from the inside out. Or you can choose to step up to the plate and make a positive lifestyle change.

Start making whole food choices, and quickly you'll begin experiencing what healthy eating's all about.
When you're pondering different whole foods, just think about foods that are closest to their natural state. A baked potato is a whole food, French fries are NOT! Just to be certain, here's a list of some whole foods you may or may not have thought about.

Examples Whole Foods
*Fresh fruits and vegetables
*Fresh herbs
*Grains - wheat, oats, rice, barley, corn, and spelt
*Unpasteurized milk and milk products
*Free-Range meats void of chemicals, preservatives, hormones, and medicines

NOTE: The further grains go along in the refining process, the less likely they're going to be classified as a *whole* food. The more processed they are the, less nutrition they have.

My Thoughts . . .
Understanding what whole foods are is important in establishing a solid base from which to build and implement your healthy eating strategy. There is a difference between organic and whole foods. But both are your best route to good health, less disease, and greater energy. The choice is yours to make.

Benefits of Eating Whole Foods

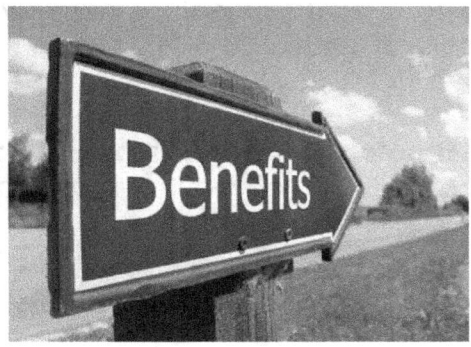

The more we dig past the surface of nutrition and healthy eating, the more sense it makes to eat the way our ancestors did hundreds of years ago. Fueling their bodies with all-natural wholesome foods straight from nature, void of harmful processing, chemicals and preservatives, that are scientifically proven to interfere with good health mentally and physically.

It's not always practical to eat whole foods. But the idea is not to be perfect. Just aim to consume whole foods as much as possible. This is beneficial to your body and mind on so many levels.

Eating whole food means:

*Choosing whole grains instead of processed and refined - *brown instead of white*

*Filling your plate full of fresh fruits, vegetables, and wholesome beans, instead of depending on supplementation - *the real deal instead of pill popping*

*Smoothie drinks made with fresh fruits and vegetables, not store juice or sugared slush drinks - *natural instead of processed sugars*

*Grilled free-range chicken instead of deep fried chicken nuggets - *natural meats void of hormones and other chemicals, instead of high fat chicken with less nutrients and oodles of additives*

*Baked sweet potato instead of a bag of potato chips - *all natural complex carbohydrates, instead of nutritionless processed simple carbohydrates*

*Dish of fresh fruit unsweetened, instead of a fruit pastry - *loads of natural vitamins and minerals, instead of processed high fat, calorie loaded, and no nutrient sweets*

*Green tea instead of soda - *natural beverages with numerous health benefits, instead of a big glass of sugar that gives you a hyper high, and sets you up for a depressing fall*

*Apple or pear, instead of a fruit snack - *whole and healthy simple carbohydrate with energy and nutrient rich sugars, instead of processed fruit snacks with lots of sugars, additives, and little nutritional value*

Annemarie Colbin, Ph.D, of Food and Healing, states eating more natural whole foods is your direct route to better health, more energy, less fat, disease avoidance. Choosing fresh fruits and vegetables, whole grains, legumes and nuts, are fantabulous whole foods choices cuz they've got plenty of fiber and nutrients, often lost in processing. Phytochemicals are one of the victims.
Whole food eating is beginning to make a comeback. Music to everyone's ears!

Let's have a gander at a few reasons whole foods should be making their way to your belly:

Nutrient Advantage

Experts report, a large portion of the population gets too little Vitamin C and A, potassium, fiber, and magnesium to start. Disease studies show people who get adequate amounts of these vitamins and minerals in specific, lower their risk considerably of developing heart disease, high blood pressure and cholesterol, diabetes, and cancer.

Of course whole food eating tops up your stores, and ensures you're level on the nutrient playing field.
The majority of missing nutrients in your diet can simply be rectified with a **whole food - plant based** eating strategy.

Essential Phytochemicals

What are Phytochemicals? They're chemical substances naturally found in plants that aim to prevent free radicals from manifesting within your body and producing disease through cell damage. Scientists are discovering new phytochemicals regularly, and right now there are more than 1,000 known.

If you want phytochemicals, you need to eat plant-based foods in their natural state. Processing them often zaps their disease-preventing benefits.

Lycopene is found in red colored phytochemical, in foods like tomatoes and red peppers.

Anthocyanins give the marvelous blue color to berries. *Pterostilbene* is a powerful antioxidant that seems to trigger the cells in berries and grapes to metabolize fat and cholesterol.

In order to take advantage of these protective chemicals, you'll need to fill your body full of whole foods.

Healthy Fats

Trans fats and saturated fats are what you need to steer clear of when healthy eating is our focus. Processed and packaged foods are loaded with these *bad* fats, making it very difficult to lose weight, and program your body to develop disease.

Whole foods have very little if any *bad* fat. They have healthy fats in moderate amounts, which is exactly what your body requires to find that perfect balance of maintaining energy, and metabolizing nasty fat.

Good fats also help with deterring disease and improving brain function. Unsaturated fats like sunflower oil, avocado, and olive oil, should be your fats of choice for optimal health.

Wholesome Fiber

Wholesome fiber is abundant in most whole foods. Where it's lost in processed foods.

US Good and Drug Administration recommends between 20 and 30 grams of fiber per day.
Infamous Dr. Mercola says fiber benefits your health by:
*Improving blood sugar control
*Stabilizing weight
*Making you feel full faster
*Lower the risk of diabetes and heart disease
*Moves your GI tract along
*Fiber feeds on pathogenic bacteria, healing gut issues
*Aids in digestion
*Boots crappy toxins out of your system
*Supports skin health
*Contributes to heart health

Ridding your body of harmful toxins is an essential preventative measure toward great health. Whole foods eating is a fantabulous start.

Whole Grains
Whole grain foods not only have loads of fiber, but they also have so many nutrients vital to great health. Switching to whole grain foods lowers your risk of developing diabetes, lowers cholesterol, and blood pressure.

Adipose tissue - the fat tissue around your organs and muscles - is shown in lower levels when people chose whole grains over refined.

Less "Extras"
Whole foods don't have preservatives, chemicals, or harmful hormones added. The *extras* that allow processed foods to last so long on the shelf, and taste so sugary sweet.

These *extras* make foods addictive, and easily to form into bad habit. Eating whole foods eliminates the harmful *extras* that directly trigger disease, and interfere with good health.

Other Benefits of Whole Foods
Reduce the risk of cataracts, which is a clouding over of the lens of the eye found in over half of people over 75

Reduces the amino acid homocysteine, which is often accumulated to high levels in people that don't eat healthy. This increases the risk of cardiovascular disease and stroke

*Healthy isoflavones and lignans are **phytonutrients**, found in whole foods like berries and flaxseed. Research* *studies show phytonutrients lower the risk for cancers of the reproductive system.*

TAKE ACTION! Tips for Incorporating Whole Foods into Your Life

Choose 100% Whole Grain
*When it comes to whole grains, breads and starches, choose 100% whole grains without preservatives. Natural whole grains spoil faster without additives. If bread lasts up to two weeks, it's got crap added.
However, if a *whole grain* bread expires in a few days, chances are pretty good it's full of whole grain goodness. Be sure to read the label to be sure.

Snack on Fresh Fruits and Veggies
*If your tummy is grumbling for a snack, grab fresh fruits and vegetables. Always have them prepped and ready in the fridge, so when you're tummy's rumbling, you don't have to worry about cutting them up.

Often that's just enough of a deterrent to set your sites on the snack cupboard.
Filling your plate at mealtime with plenty of sweet and tasty veggies is also important. The fiber fills you up and helps blast fat. The antioxidants protect you from disease, and give you ample energy to keep your body and mind strong, and disease away.

Substitute Flour
*If you're a baker, you can start substituting whole grain flour for traditional white. Begin with half and half, cuz some recipes don't fare so well with all whole grain. Better yet, start switching to nutrient rich all-natural whole grain recipes. Often they're tastier anyway. Change is good!

Cut Back on Processed
*Scale back on the high fat, little nutrients, calorie loaded processed, and packaged, convenience foods. These foods fill your body and blood full of harmful fat. Slowing down internal system function, stressing your body, and zapping your confidence.

Go For Beans
*Try and eat more beans as snacks and with meals. They are full of fiber, plant protein, heart healthy phytochemicals, and numerous other essential nutrients. Beans help build lean muscle, and fuel your body for long-term energy that lasts. Beans are flavorful, inexpensive, and versatile.

Adzuki Beans are little sweet red beans that are easy on the digestive system, and taste fantabulous with brown rice and celery, for excellent protein and fiber-rich patties.

Chick peas are used often in the heart-healthy Mediterranean Diet. They're great for taming potent spices; adding to chili, soups, and salads.

Kidney Beans are popular in chili, casseroles, soups, salads, and stir fry's. Just be sure to fully cook them, otherwise they're nasty tooth-breaking hard.

Those are just a few examples of how you can use tasty, nutrient, and fiber dense beans to your advantage.

Did You Know?
Tongues of Fire and **Mortgage Lifters** are a few of the crazy named beans available throughout the United States!
My Thoughts . . .

It's fair to say the benefit of whole food plant based eating is endless. Technically we should shoot for 100% percent whole food eating, but that's just not practical.

We all lead hectic lives, full of daily stresses, and gynormous limitations with time.

WE LOVE CONVENIENCE!
Unfortunately grabbing unhealthy processed fast foods seems to be the norm. Turning into habit quickly. And it doesn't take long for you to have an unhealthy, energy stealing, fat fueling, disease triggering, and habit to break.

Science says, whole foods are best. Medical professionals agree.

And if you're a natural troublemaker looking for conflict. Good luck finding a health and wellness expert that isn't on board with wholesome and healthy whole food eating!

What Nutrients Do Plants Provide?

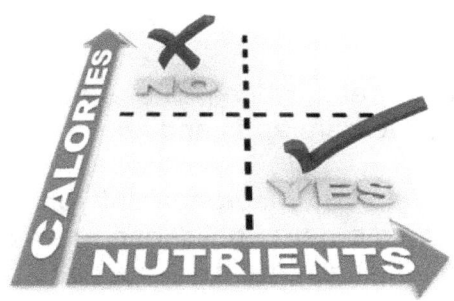

In order to be healthy and happy, with a body the super sexy-strong-fit-healthy, and a mind that's sharp and clear, you need specific nutrients.

The six basic nutrients your body needs are:
*Carbohydrates
*Protein
*Fat
*Vitamins
*Minerals
*Water

Carbohydrates are required for energy, breaking down protein, and for protecting your body from harmful toxins. You need complex carbohydrates, cuz the glucose pro-vided is critical to good health.

Whole grains and vegetables are great sources. With starch as an important component in the big picture of fantabulous health.

Servings - 6-8/day
Avoiding high sugar, high fat, simple refined sugar carbohydrates, with very little nutrients, is important.

Sources: White bread, white pasta and rice, pastries, cookies, chocolate bars and candy

Protein is an important macronutrient your body needs in large quantities, in order to build lean muscle, regulate hormones, fight disease, repair tissue, and provide energy.

Protein is essential because it isn't manufactured by the body, nor is it stored. This means you need to consume it daily. Your body needs 22 amino acids in order to produce protein, and it's only got 14 naturally. You've got to eat diverse complete proteins to get the other 8.

Sources: Various meats, fish, chicken, dairy products, eggs, nuts, beans, and quinoa

Note: *When choosing lean meats for whole food eating, you should look for meats that are void of hormones, antibiotics, or other drugs. And the animals should be fed an organic diet that steers clear of pesticides and other harmful toxins. Au natural is what you're looking for.*

Servings - 2-3/day
Fat is something you simply can't live without. The two basic types are saturated and unsaturated. Fat provides more energy than both macronutrients protein, and car-

bohydrates. It helps with vitamin absorption, keeps you warm, levels temperature, and protects your vital organs. Saturated fats like butter and lard, interfere with your good health, and contribute to obesity and serious disease when consumed in large amounts. Trans fat is even more dangerous than saturated, because it's chemically altered so food has more flavor, stability, and a longer shelf life to start.

Processed foods often have these NAUGHTY fats.
Sources of GOOD fats: Avocado, olive oil, sunflower oil, and olive oil

Servings - Most of us don't need to worry about getting enough fat in our diet, but focus on eating good fats not bad ones, along with cutting back. Less than 30% of your daily caloric intake should come from fats. No more than 10% should come from saturated fats.

Vitamins are chemicals your body required to process vital nutrients, build genes, red bloods cells, proteins and hormones, and regulate your central nervous system. By eating a diverse diet filled with plenty of fresh fruits and vegetables, lean meats, low fat dairy products, and complex carbohydrates you should be able to provide your body with adequate amounts of vitamins to maintain optimal health.

Sources: Poultry, fish, dairy, lean meat, eggs, fruits and vegetables

Minerals help keep your body and mind strong. These are inorganic substances your body required for making bones, teeth, body fluid regulation, generating blood cells, and assisting in natural chemical processes. There are two main types of essential minerals; macronutrients and micronutrients.

Macronutrients include protein, carbohydrates and fat.

Micronutrients, which the body needs in small amounts, include zinc, copper, cobalt, iron, iodine, manganese, fluoride, molybdenum, and selenium.

Eating a healthy well balanced diet should provide adequate amounts of micronutrients.

Water is hands down the most important component for your body. Up to 75% of your body is water. 6-8 glasses a day of pure, natural and tasty water, is required for smooth internal bodily system function.

Water purges toxins from your body, maintains skin, nails and hair, aids digestion, and transports vital nutrients throughout your body via the bloodstream. Water hydrates and gives you energy to function throughout the day.

If you don't get enough water, you'll become dehydrating. Leaving you fatigued, lethargic, and in extreme cases, confused in thought.

Of course if you're exercising regularly, your body's burning more energy, and needs more water. Keep in mind, there's a difference between a soda and glass of water. Your best choices to drink are water, herbal teas, and clear soups. Sodas are just full of excess sugars, directly linked to obesity and disease.

Servings - 6-8 glasses/day to start
Now you've got the basic idea of what your body needs to survive.
Where to plants fit in?
Plants and Carbohydrates

28

Plants provide your body with the macronutrients and micronutrients it needs to function optimally. Plant-based foods, including bananas, sweet potatoes, apples, pears and spinach, are quite high in carbs. More than protein or fat.

Since carbohydrates are the main source of energy for your cells, it's important you get enough carbs into your diet.

According to the *American Nutrition Center*, up to 65% of your caloric intake should come from carbohydrate sources. This is easily attainable through whole food options.

Plants and Protein
If you're eating animal foods like meat, eggs and dairy products, you'll give your body complete proteins. So your body gets all 20 essential amino acids in one shot.

VEGAN NOTE - You can give your body all the protein it requires without using animal products, but you're going to have to combine various foods. Simply because none of these plant-based foods have complete proteins, providing each of the 20 amino acids.

The exception to the rules is quinoa. A complete protein that's plant based.

It's definitely harder, but certainly isn't impossible to put the pieces of this protein puzzle together without complete protein sources.

Just means you need to eat a variety of protein rich plant foods throughout the day to make sure you get your protein. An example might be eating some brown rice or pasta at lunch and having some chick peas at dinner.

Perhaps you want to have some legumes for a snack and a handful of nuts after dinner. Diversity is key here and so long as you are eating a wide variety of colorful and protein rich plant-based foods daily you will keep on top of your bodily protein needs.

Quinoa is an exception to the rule. It is the only complete protein that is plant based.

Experts agree that up to 35% of your daily calories should come from protein.

Fiber and Plants
Fiber is one component of healthy eating you don't have to worry about lacking with plants. Plants are loaded with healthy fiber that regulates your bodily systems, naturally removing toxic buildup by eliminating waste. This means your body's going to function with more gusto.

There are two main types of fiber; soluble and insoluble.

Soluble fiber comes mainly from oats and fruits, and helps slow your digestive process down, making you feel fuller longer. It also allows for better nutrient absorption.

Insoluble fiber is abundant in natural veggies and grains. It helps increase the speed of digestion, pushing waste out faster, and keeping your internal systems functioning smoothly.

Nutritionists suggest about 15 grams of fiber for each thousand calories consumed is adequate.

Plants and Minerals

Plants offer all sorts of important minerals you need each day. Minerals are simply non-living substances that infiltrate into plants through the soil.

Magnesium is plentiful in legumes and whole grains, necessary for nerve and muscle function.

Phosphorus is found in various nuts and beans, helping to strengthen tissues and bones. Potassium is abundant in bananas, regulating electrolytes, and supporting cellular fluid function, important in heart and muscle function and regulation.

Vitamins and Plants
Vitamins are living and made by plants. Vitamins are a must to maintain good health. *Vitamin A* is found in leafy green veggies, helping to keep your eyes healthy. Broccoli, strawberries and oranges are loaded with *Vitamin C*, strengthening your immune systems to start. Healthy whole grains are loaded with heart healthy *B Vitamins*, and gather energy from the macronutrients to help your internal systems function effectively.

My Thoughts . . .
With knowledge and an open mind, you can definitely get all the essential nutrients your body requires from a Whole Foods Plant Based Diet. In doing so, you're choosing to fuel your body naturally without the interference harmful processing serves up.

Energy levels rise, fat disappears, thinking gets crisper, chronic symptoms lessen or disappear, and disease is avoided. **Prevention** *is key to fantabulous health, and choosing to stick with Mother Nature when fueling your body, pushes your great health straight up to the top!*

Sample Eating

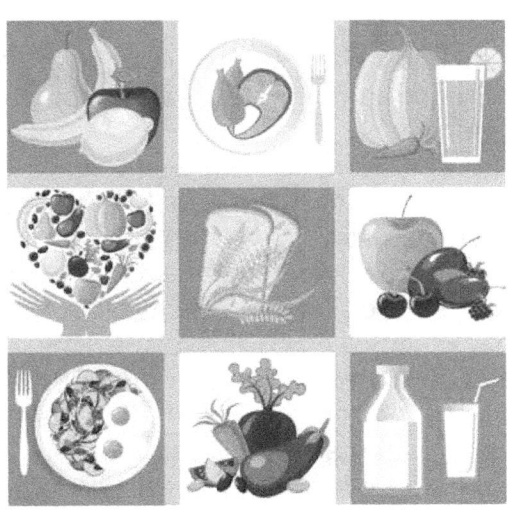

If you didn't know this already, your health and wellness, your life attitude, life decisions, energy levels, positivity and quality of life, ARE dependent on how you fuel your body.

The foods you choose to eat, in what quantity and when, are all factors dictating how you're going to look, feel, act, think, and perceive life.

Choosing natural energizing whole foods when you can, helps communicate to your mind and body, that you care about yourself. That you're looking to make the most of life. And understand a strong body void of disease, and a clear mind that's sharp and effective, are MUSTS in the game of life. If you don't take care of your mental and physical, they aren't going to take care of you.

RUN FROM THE BAD!

Avoiding convenient processed and packaged nutrient-poor foods is absolute in healthy Whole Foods Plant Based Diet eating. Plenty of fresh fruits and vegetables, whole grains, nuts, lean meats, fish, poultry, legumes, and eggs, are smart options. Providing your body with all the nutrients required to stay lean and strong, excited to stand for tomorrow!

Whole food choices and getting back with nature and pure goodness, is a step in the right direction. Don't expect to be perfect. It's just important to do your best to make wholesome food choices always.

Drink Note - Ensure you carry a bottle of pure water around with you. It's important you get 6-8 glasses of water each day. You can also include green tea, herbal teas, and natural fruit infused waters. The latter is just slicing up your favorite fruits and putting them in a jug of water in the fridge the night before.

Overnight the flavors infuse into the water. This makes a delicious all-natural beverage to make water a little more exciting. Stay away from caffeinated drinks, sodas and fruit juices that are loaded with sugars, additives, and no nutrients.

Here are a few sample meals that'll help you transition your mind and actions towards healthier and wholesome.

Breakfast

It's the most important meal of the day. Your body has been on autopilot all night, and is depleted of essential vitamins and minerals, the vital nutrients it needs to function optimally.

Eating a wholesome, healthy breakfast BEFORE you set foot out the door, needs to be practice and practiced again, until it becomes habit. There's no room for excuses.

Choice One
Instead of having a boxed cereal breakfast or package of quick ready oats, start your day with an omelet of free-range eggs, fresh herbs, spinach, tomato, onion, peppers, and Parmesan cheese.

You'll need foods that are natural and wholesome. Foods that were around back in the day, when your ancestors were eating so healthy and natural. These foods provide just the right amount of healthy fats that aren't going to add fat to your frame, but help your body better absorb all the vitamins and minerals it requires to shine.

Choice Two
How about a dish of whole unpasteurized yogurt with loads of fresh berries and sprinkled with almonds? This provides the protein and good carbs your body needs to build lean muscle, increase your metabolism, or rate in which you burn fat, and starve off disease, with those protective antioxidants from fresh berries.

Of course almonds also provide you with just enough fat to give you energy and help your thinking stay sharp.

Lunch and Supper
What many people don't realize, is that your body works best on a schedule. It likes to know when you'll be eating

for the most part, so it can adjust what it needs to accomplish accordingly.

Skipping meals and starving your body is all wrong. This is what screws up the smooth running of your internal systems, short-circuits your brain, and causes negative interference that'll give you loads of illness and disease, both mental and physical.

Intermittent eating mucks up your sleep schedule, triggers anxiety, turns off your natural fat burning hormones, and makes you lazy and tired. Not eating will drop your blood sugar levels down dangerously low, so that when you do eat, particularly if you're eating junk, your sugar levels will shoot straight to the top.

This ping-pong action has proven to trigger diabetes, or at least increase your risk. Not to mention nastier mood swings, and a complete rewiring of your system to muck you up.

Do yourself a favor. Listen to your body and eat when it needs it. Next, make sure you give it whole foods so it can get the job done This helps you to look fantastic, feel great, and have ample energy on tap!

Making sure you fuel your body with lean protein, vegetables and good fat, sets your body up to smile.

Choice One
For lunch, have a spinach salad with grilled free-range chicken, tomato, cucumber, onion, sesame seeds, sunflowers seeds, and a drizzle of coconut oil-based dressing.

For dinner, grill a salmon steak with a drizzle of olive oil and fresh herbs, grilled sweet potato, sliced avocado, and steamed broccoli, kale, carrots, peas, beans, and water chestnuts.

Natural organic whole grain bread goes nicely with this.

Choice Two
For lunch, try placing a cup of quinoa into a Romaine leaf for a wrap. You can add tomato and cucumber. A cup of unpasteurized whole yogurt with sliced banana, mango, and crushed almonds tops it off perfectly.

For dinner, grill a chicken breast drizzled in soybean oil and fresh herbs. Steam parsnip, broccoli, spinach, peppers, eggplant, and lentils, for a nutritious side loaded with protein for calorie burning, carbs for long-lasting energy, and essential vitamins and minerals to support your internal systems and their function.

Snacking
Unfortunately, we're conditioned to view snacking as devilish, sneaky, and unhealthy. Snacking is often choosing processed sweet foods, high in bad fat, sugars and calories, and have very little nutritional gain. This includes chips, cookies, muffins, French fries, chocolate bars, and other sweets.

These food choices blast us with short-lived energy, because of the massive dose of sugar. They also leave you hungrier lickety-split!

Here are a few excellent whole food options to wrap your head around, that'll give you the energy you're searching for, and the staying power that makes it *sweet*.

Handful of nuts and dried fruit (careful not to overdose because a serving is 2-3 tbsp.), gives you the protein and good fats your mind and body needs

Hardboiled eggs and raw veggies, gives you protein, iron, and the fiber, your body needs to naturally get rid of toxic buildup

Celery and all-natural peanut butter, delivers fiber, protein for energy, and good fats in perfect combination

Sliced avocado on fresh fruit and veggies, provides healthy fats, protein, carbohydrates, and vitamins and minerals, to help build your body and mind strong

Fruit salad with plenty of berries, talk about a protective punch

Handful of raisins and organic kale chips, vitamins and minerals to energize

Sliced sweet potato crisps, slice sweet potatoes, sprinkle with herbs and back until crisp

All-natural beef jerky will give your body a quick dose of protein without the fuss

All-natural fruit juice smoothie made with almond milk, dates, and fruits of your choice, fat metabolizing energy with staying power

My Thoughts . . .
Whole food eating doesn't have to be difficult. In fact it's our high-tech fast food eating that is causing all the ruckus. Taking the time to "tell" yourself all the positives of eating whole foods, is your first step in the transformation process.

Set yourself up for success by trying something you can see yourself enjoying. In other words, consider your pref- erences and tolerances in all food choices, and open your mind to change.

One step at a time, and allow yourself to take a step backwards here and there. You're only human.
You never know unless you try. And by using these meal and snack ideas as a guide, you'll find what works for your body mentally and physical. This approach has to be married, or it just won't work.

Disease Prevention and Whole Food Connection

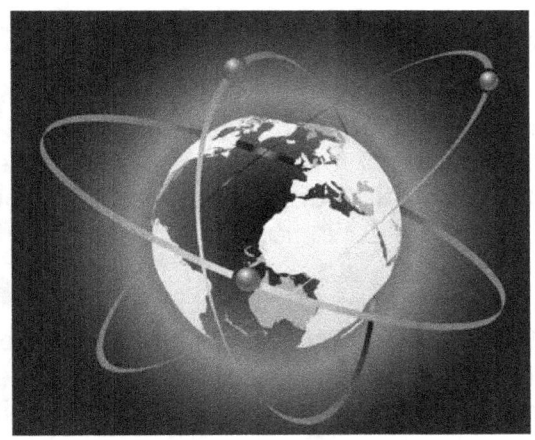

Why is it important you eat healthier by choosing natural whole foods?

*Prevents bone and muscle loss and vitamin deficiency that will result in serious disease and chronic conditions

*Disease prevention including cancer, stroke, cardiovascular disease, diabetes, and osteoporosis to start

*Naturally lowers high blood pressure, the risk for celiac disease, and diabetes

In order to maintain good health you've got to give your body all the macro and micronutrients it requires. If you survive on processed fast foods, there's **ZERO** chance you'll stay healthy. It's only a matter of time before you

41

trigger illness and disease that will eventually take your life.

Adequate amounts of protein, carbohydrates, fats, vitamins, minerals, and water, are critical in keeping your organs and internal systems functioning optimally. This includes the health of your mind, because if your physical isn't healthy, your mind is truly mucked up.

Take note, vitamins and minerals come from all-natural substances necessary for your good health. They're essential for physical function, thinking, and the metabolic process that breaks down flabby fat.

Disease Prevention and Control
PREVENTION is everything in life. Just think about it from a practical perspective. If you happen to be goofing off and break your leg, you can get it *fixed*, but it's still never going to be the same.

Regardless of how skilled the surgeon was setting your bone, or how fantabulous your physical therapist was, your leg will never be as healthy or strong as it was. A break is a break.

Means your leg is weaker than it was before you broke it up, even after it's completely healed. As years go by, your break may come back and bug you because of chronic aches and pains, or perhaps the break was bad enough that it threw off your bodily alignment, causing you to favor one side. Over time, this may develop into a limp, and the side effects snowball from there.

Same thing applies with disease. If you can prevent disease with healthy and energizing whole food choices, why wouldn't you?

Do you want to have symptoms after the fact for the rest of your life?

Wouldn't you rather make the changes now, so you don't ever have to experience heart disease, stroke, diabetes, or any other sickness?

Experts agree, whole food eating is the best choice you can make for your body. It's all about perspective here, give and take. You don't have to be perfect and make a whole food choice **EVERY** time.

The idea is to re-teach yourself how to eat. Eventually you're going to **WANT** to eat an apple instead of a bag of potato chips. A grilled chicken with steamed asparagus and cauliflower will make your mouth water, instead of a greasy burger and fries.

It's all about **DECIDING** to make a change for the better, and committing to it. It's setting yourself up for success, practicing and giving it time to sink in. You **CAN** do it if you want.

Would you agree that obesity is the root of most evil and preventable disease?
Scientists agree that losing weight, even just a few pounds, greatly reduces your risk of developing all sorts of serious disease. By simply choosing to eat less high-energy-dense foods and more low-energy-dense foods, you're increasing the ability for your body to burn fat and lose weight.

High-energy-dense foods are processed foods, fried foods, sweets, full fat salad dressings, and other devilish delights. They're often loaded with saturated fats and high cholesterol, which mucks up your health.

BEST MOVE - Lower calorie foods with ample nutrients is what you want to load your body with. And this is what you'll find with low-energy-dense food options. Low-energy-dense foods are healthy choices including fresh vegetables and fruit.

The *Dietary Guide for Americans* suggests a healthy whole food diet should consist of:
*Focusing on fresh fruits and vegetables, whole grains, and milk products

*Adequate amounts of lean meats, fish, skinless chicken and turkey, nuts, eggs, and beans

*Include sparing amounts of healthy unsaturated fats.

Choose low in cholesterol, and avoid saturated and Trans fat as much as possible. Also avoid added sugars and sodium.

Disease prevention **BEGINS** with fueling your body right. Which also helps naturally remove toxic buildup from your system, triggering disease and illness. Processed and packaged foods have chemicals and preservatives your body doesn't know how to flush from your system. Over time they build up and interferes with good health. Choosing whole foods and drinking plenty of water, is a natural to give your body the nutrients it requires to fight disease, and the liquid and fiber necessary to purge toxins.

Fabulous Disease Fighting Whole Foods
Fatty Fish
In fatty fish like tuna and salmon, you'll find omega 3 fatty acids. They help naturally lower blood fats, preventing blood clots from developing. It's these blood clots that are a symptom of heart disease.

44

Studies show having fatty fish twice a week lowers your risk of heart disease tremendously.

Sweet Potato
Sweet potatoes are loaded with protective antioxidants, beta-carotene, E and C vitamins, folate, iron, copper, calcium, and potassium. There are nice quantities of fiber that encourage a healthy digestive system, and the protective antioxidants prevent cancer and cardiovascular disease.

Various Nuts
Nuts are tasty treats that give your body the healthy fat it requires to function optimally. This fat helps lower cholesterol naturally, which is a trigger for a variety of serious diseases.

Nuts also have plenty of:
*Fiber
*Protein
*E and A vitamins
*Selenium
Nuts are a great energy dense snack to hold you over. But you've got to be careful, because they're very high in calories and good fat. A handful is lots for a serving.

Eggs
Eggs are one of the best sources of protein, and have essential vitamins and minerals necessary for good eye health. The choline in eggs is an important nutrient, particularly for pregnant women. Eggs are easy to eat, and fit into any meal in moderation.

An egg a day keeps the doctor away.

Spinach, Romaine and Others Greens

Your best whole foods to deter disease are a wide array of leafy green veggies. Packed full of minerals, essential vitamins, vitamin C, magnesium, phytochemicals, antioxidants, iron, folate, fiber, and so much more.
It makes sense to load your plate up.

Experts suggest eating a diet with magnesium helps lower your risk of developing diabetes. Spinach has lots of magnesium.

My Thoughts . . .
In general, fruits and vegetables are the powerhouses *of disease fighting and prevention nutrients, some of which are an array of minerals, vitamins, fiber, antioxidants, and phytochemicals.*

Ensuring you get at least 5-6 servings a day, helps lower your risk of cancer and numerous other diseases. Choosing to bypass processed foods and throwing refined eating out the window, is a wise-owl smart move. Replacing it with whole food plant based eating, gives your body and mind a fighting chance.
The choice as always is yours.

Exercising and Whole Foods

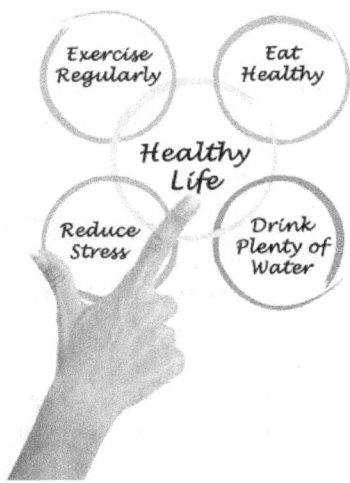

Do you want to exercise with your tank half empty or full to the brim?

Would you prefer clean pure energy that lasts, or intermittent bursts of highs and lows when exercising?

If you eat foods loaded with harmful fats, sugars and calories, you won't exercise effectively and efficiently, to burn off pesky fat stores. Processed fast foods, pastries and sweets, give your body **FAST** energy that disappears as quickly as it came.

This energy is not useful for the body. It's the wrong fuel to convert into energy, to maximize fat burn and increase energy.

If you want to increase your metabolism by exercising AND burn off stored fat, you need to give your body adequate amounts of good fat, lean protein, and complex carbohydrates.

These macronutrients don't come from nutrition-less fast foods, that are fried and come in boxes. You need to build lean muscle to burn fat. And if you're building muscle with exercising, you need oodles of lean protein.

Before and After Exercising
You should have a snack with protein and complex carbohydrates, to provide the easily accessible fast nutrition your body needs, to build lean muscle and zap fat.

VIP - Be sure to always drink plenty of water. This ensures the essential macronutrients, vitamins and minerals, get dispersed throughout your body, for maximized energy and results.
This is also important after you've finished exercising, because you need to replenish your vitamin stores.

Sample Snacks
*Apples dipped in all-natural peanut butter are a perfect protein and carbohydrate-rich snack, to give your body the energy it requires to exercise. A whole grain bagel with peanut butter also works nicely about an hour before training, and immediately after.

*All-natural energy bars that are 70% carbohydrates and 30% protein, are also an excellent choice. Be sure you don't choose one with excess sugar added.

*Fresh veggies and hummus are perfect energizers when exercising. The vegetables give you fiber, carbohydrates, and antioxidant protection. While protein storage is taken care of with the hummus. About half a cup of hummus with about a cup of veggies should do the trick.

*If you're really in a pinch, a handful of nuts should do the trick. This gives your body fast access to easily absorbed protein, omega-3s, vitamin E, selenium, and your carb needs are satisfied too.

*Tossing a grilled chicken breast in a Romaine lettuce leaf, with about a 1/4 cup of quinoa is tasty, and it gives your body and mind the energy to perform. This can be eaten cold, and works really well as leftovers.

*Peanut butter and banana on whole grain bread or crackers, is another snack that packs a punch. You should use a 1-2 tbsp. of peanut butter, half a banana, and one piece of whole grain bread or 6-8 crackers.

Your body's a machine that's dependent on a wide array of nutrients to function optimally. If you deprive your body of what it needs to formulate new cells, repair damaged ones, work all your internal organs, and ensure all the receptors in your body are working well, you'll run into trouble in time.

Usually your body grabs attention with aches, pains, and disease. We usually ignore it, and let it manifest into something permanent, which takes away from our quality of life.

The choice is yours.
How much should you exercise?
Of course this is a subjective question. But most experts agree people should do some sort of exercising every day. What's more important, is setting yourself up for success, because something is better than nothing.

Always consider your preferences and tolerances prior to starting.

30-45 minutes of moderate to intense cardiovascular activity, 3-5 days a week is a great place to start. Add to that 2-3 days of strength training, or weight lifting for 15 minutes each time, and you should be good to go.

Honestly, it really doesn't take a whole lot of time to keep your body in shape physically, IF you commit to exercising smart.

HAPPY FACT - You don't have to be a gym rat to get physically healthy.
Find the activities you enjoy!

If you can't stand going to the gym then, maybe you want to ride your bike, and lift some light weights at home? Perhaps swimming is something you love? If you enjoy classes, a boot camp training session three times a week, for an hour each time, is all you need to get fit! These classes maximize the energy you burn, and are probably one of the *best* forms of exercise out there.

Why?
Boot camp session use an interval training method that keeps your mind and body guessing. Which means you're never going to get bored, and both physically and mentally are always challenged.

Boot camp sessions challenge you each class to dig deeper. You're in competition with yourself amongst a group of varying skill levels. These classes' alternate periods of high intensity and low intensity cardiovascular, muscular, and stretching and toning exercising, while keeping your heart rate up and fat burning off.

It's the diversity of these sessions that make them so effective. Exercises are always changing, along with intensity, weight, reps, duration, pace, and pattern. You might as well make the most of your exercise time right? You run on other people's energy, because everyone pushes to do their very best. Fat loss, lean muscle gain, and a beautiful toned and healthy body is the result. It's pretty tough not to get caught up in the positive adrenaline when it surrounds you!

The best part of all, is you work at your level always, and it's the instructors that continuously push and inspire you to try harder each time. This means more fat loss, improved self-confidence, and a leaner, stronger, and happier you.

Eating a well- balanced diet with the right amount of protein, carbohydrates, good fat, and vitamins and minerals, is a smarty-pants move. Add plenty of pure water, and you'll set your body up to burn fat, build lean muscle, and feel like a million bucks; mind, body, and soul.

My Thinking . . .
Without a healthy physical *body you're sunk. Every single thing you do is dependent on being physically able. Even if you want to smile, you've got to use your facial muscles and mind to do so.*

This takes energy, and means your body needs to use up some of the energy you've given it. This energy needs to be replenished. And when you're exercising, you really need to pay attention, because you're using more energy in the form of protein, carbohydrates, and fats, to give your body the ability to work hard for you.

If the energy isn't there, and you're still trying to exercise, stress is triggered, and this negatively affects you.

Did you know that if you're training and don't get enough protein for your body to use for muscle formation and bodily function, it'll break down muscle for energy? You've got to get your lean protein daily!

If you want to burn off fat, you have to eat. Make sure your body's got enough lean protein and complex carbohydrates, to give your body the ability to burn fat off. When your body is fueled optimally, all you've got to worry about is actually implementing the physical exercise. Your body will take care of the rest.

Your body is uniquely complex. And it's in your best interest, to eat healthy. Whole food eating in the right combinations, sets you up to build your body lean, while keeping your energy levels happy and high. Once again, the choice is yours.

Whole Foods and the Mental Benefits

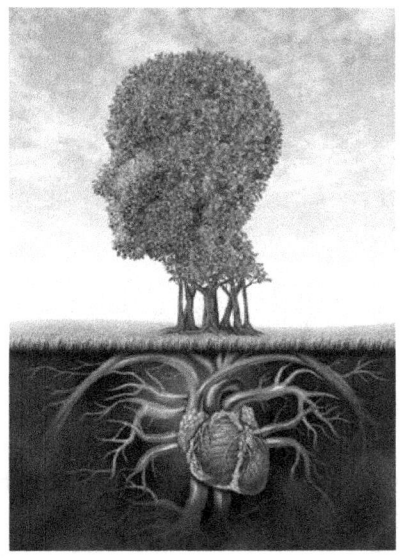

When it comes to getting healthy, we often focus solely on the physical. Many people assume if you're in shape physically, that you're healthy. This just isn't the case. Your good health is dependent on both physical and mental. You can't really have one without the other.

Underrated Fact - Your mind is a powerful thing. It controls your reality, how you perceive life in general, and whether or not you're going to commit to getting healthy for life and feel great about it, or quit.

It's your mind that dictates your actions. Making sure your *mental,* or *thinking* is optimal, only helps you reach your goals faster and more effectively.

What good is it to have a six pack and have He-man physically strength, if you're always depressed and un-happy with you?

Is it so overwhelming you stay inside your house most days?

Making healthy whole food choices will help, by encour-aging your mind and body to function as one, which is necessary for optimal health.

Fact: It goes without saying, that your diet directly affects your mood.

Your diet also affects how you act and your internal brain function. If you aren't eating well, your energy levels are likely see-sawing, on top of the world one minute and de-pressingly devastated the next.

If you're choosing to eat junk food meals you'll rarely be satisfied for long. Loads of sugars and unhealthy fats dif-fuse into your system in large doses, leaving you hungry and unsatisfied all the time. And because of the pre-servatives and harmful chemical interference, you're going to have all sorts of troubles. From sleep issues, to skin breakouts, extreme fatigue, and emotional chaos. In how your see yourself, your life attitude, passions, and ability to think clearly, and with effectiveness.

Food is oodles important in your big picture health. According to *Dietitians of Canada,* healthy eating pro-motes mental health by enhancing food security, social inclusion, self-trust, and positive body image, while minimizing health and social inequities.

Understanding which foods are best not only for your physical well- being, but also your mental, is top priority. You're worth it!

Nutritional factors influencing your emotional well-being

*Protein intake
*Carbohydrate intake
*Fat intake
*Vitamins, minerals and alcohol intake
*Total amount of energy you take in
*Genetic composition and medical status

Even if you're missing a single vitamin, your brain function may be negatively affected.

Examples of how your eating habits affect mood
*Highs and lows of blood sugar levels
*Not getting enough vitamins and minerals, or fatty acids, can disturb your thinking
*The foods you eat, directly affect your brain function
*Specific nutrients missing, can directly affect your ability to digest food and convert it into energy
*Breathing in unclear air, interferes with brain and physical function
*Preservatives, bad fats, and other harmful chemicals added to food, can affect your brain, manifest over time, and create disease

One deadly habit that affects far too many people, is depending on fast food eating to fuel the body. Fat foods are anything but good for your body or thinking.

They're loaded with saturated fats, calories, salt, and harmful chemicals, that'll build up over time in your internal organs, and cause issue. Lipids build up in the blood over time, increasing sugar in your blood, taxing your pancreas and liver, and increasing your risk of developing diabetes.

This sort of unhealthy eating stressing your body and mind, and slowly but surely you'll poison yourself from the inside out. Choosing not to give your body and mind the clean whole foods it craves, will come with a price.

Is this a price you want to pay?
Is your good health really worth a few fries and greasy burgers?

Mental clarity and eating
Iron
If you don't give your body enough iron, you'll feel extremely fatigued, and often ill. Not having enough iron in your bloodstream leaves you without energy, causes body stress.

 By choosing to eat healthy dark leafy green veggies, whole grains, beans, and eggs, you'll provide your body with the nutrients it depends on to get healthy mentally and physically.

Folic Acid
If you aren't getting enough folic acid, you'll feel moody, tired, not hungry, and have trouble sleeping. Women that are pregnant, have got to get ample folic acid, because it's critical in normal fetal formation, growth, and development.

Eating whole foods including beans, peas, spinach, squash, and raisins, is a fantabulous way to boost stores.

Doctors recommend pregnant women take a multivitamin with folic acid just to be sure.

Omega 3s
Omega 3 fatty acids are important for decreasing cholesterol, sharpening the mind, and preventing cardiovascular disease. Fatty fish like salmon, tuna and cod, are great sources. Experts recommend feasting on fish twice a week.

Studies show, increasing your omega 3s improves brain function.

Zinc
Zinc is found in liver, eggs, seafood, numerous veggies, and red meat. If you don't get enough zinc, irreversible neurological damage may occur. Not getting enough may lead to the jitters, grumpiness, and extreme tiredness.

B Vitamins
Too much stress, combined with excessive amounts of alcohol, interferes with B vitamin storage and use. Not enough of these vitamins transforms you really tired, grumpy, moody, and you may not be able to sleep. Eating plenty of healthy whole grains, nuts, legumes, seeds and organ meats, gives your body adequate amounts. Milk, eggs, and animals meats, are also excellent sources, according to *Women's Day*.

Selenium
In order for hormones to be synthesized, selenium is required. It also protects membranes from damage. By eating plenty of seeds, nuts, eggs, grains, and seafood, you'll offer your body adequate amounts of selenium for optimal mental and physical function

My Thoughts . . .

Your mental health is just as important as the physical in the big picture. Both are intricately connected, and don't function well separately.

Eating whole foods gives your mind and body the right amount of optimal nutrients, supplying the energy required to support your body and mind for optimal function. This means you'll have the ability to deter disease, feel, and look like a million bucks, and maybe even walk around with a skip in your step.

Final Thoughts

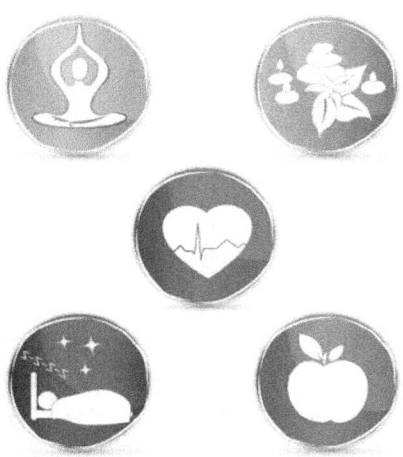

According to *Tara Gidus*, RD for the *American Dietetic Association*, whole foods eating means you're eating these foods in their natural state, loaded with vitamins, minerals, and other essential nutrients supporting optimal health.

Eating whole foods is pretty tough to argue. It's what nature Mother Nature intended. Natural, virgin, nutrient rich foods that are easily absorbed by your body. Providing the perfect energy required to function optimally mentally and physically.

SAD TRUTH - Progress and technology have messed this perfect concept up, causing harmful, and often deadly interference.

As a fast paced society, we've learnt to make habit of unhealthy processed food eating. Habits are hard to break.

Particularly when your mind and senses tell you this one tastes *really* good.

We teach our body and mind to crave sweet and nutrition-less convenience foods, and allow our emotions and life stresses to control what, when, and how much we chow down.

You routinely use things like heartache and depression, to deem valid the need for a chocolate bar, or tub of ice cream. Instead of teaching yourself to go for a run, or grab an apple. Not an apple fritter, slice of apple pie, or an apple muffin. But a real life wholesome and natural apple, picked right of the tree if possible.

People are used to this destructive cycle of habitual remorse, and just accept it as *normal*. As a lazy society unaccustomed to change, we allow overeating, obesity, and all sorts of other nasty conditions and circumstances to manifest.

On paper it seems like we just don't care.
You are in charge of you right?

SOLUTION - It's time for **YOU** to COMMIT to taking **ACTION**!
Action Steps . . .

First . . .
Acknowledge and accept change needs to happen, if you're going to get your body healthier mentally and physically.

Second . . .
Understand whole food eating is your direct route to fantabulous health.

It provides your body with the essential macronutrients and micronutrients it requires to provide energy, deter disease, burn fat, build lean muscle, and leave you feeling healthy and happy mentally, physically, spiritually, and emotionally.

Third . . .
Commit to gaining knowledge about whole foods in general. Which ones work best with your preferences and tolerances, and making sure you keep an open mind towards trying new concepts.

Fourth . . .
Make the changes necessary to start reaping the rewards. Set yourself up for success by implementing changes slowly, so they're manageable. Too much too soon, results in falling backwards into your unhealthy, but comfortable ways of days past.

Perhaps you should skip your afternoon vending machine snack, and opt for a handful of nuts, or a couple pieces of fresh fruit? Instead of having white toast with butter for breakfast, choose whole grain toast with peanut butter. It's so important you make manageable changes that make sense to you. Changes you **WANT** to commit to for life.

This isn't a fad diet that comes and goes. It's all about making changes that stick. That part's all up to you.
Go big or go home doesn't play in this park.

Fifth . . .
Actually set up your meal plans at least the day before. So you know what foods you need to buy, and you don't waste time trying to figure it out when you're hungry. That will get you into big trouble.

Sixth . . .

Experiment and figure out what sort of physical exercise fits best for your daily activity. Start off slow, and work your way forward, always checking with your healthcare provider first just to be safe.

It's so important you enjoy the exercise you choose, if you want to implement long-term. Keep in mind your best option is both diverse cardiovascular and muscle building exercises. Interval training is the golden ticket!

Seventh . . .

This one's VIP. Pinkie swear right now you'll **NEVER** quit. The only way you'll fail with the Whole Food Diet, is to actually throw in the towel. There will be setbacks, and it's important you accept this.

Most importantly, you need to accept them, let them go, and move forward. You're human and *mistakes* will happen. Onward all eyes forward is your first option.
Take the knowledge you've gained and apply it to your personal tastes, preferences, tolerances, and life beliefs. Healthy Whole foods are what Mother Nature tells us to eat.

It's really tough to re-program your thinking from what you've been taught. Technology, convenience, more money, less sleep, more *toys*, and faster cars, have slowly but surely made their way into our lives, and pushed away the basics. Like eating healthy whole foods, and entertaining ourselves with good old endorphin releasing exercise.

When stressed, go for a run instead of drowning your sorrows in a tub of double chocolate sugar loaded ice cream, while watching your favorite television program.

The price you pay for all these convenient luxuries in life is ultimately your health. That's ironic, seeing as your health is the most important asset you own.

It's time to make a natural and wholesome change for the better, one step at a time, don't you think?
You've the choice to look for the positive or the negative in life. Take the positives from this book that work for you, and go make your mind, body, and soul smile!

Life's just too short not to tune into optimism. If your glass is half full, then I invite you to read my writing, and if you have a minute to spare when you're through, **I would appreciate your review.** This will help me better myself and my writing. I thank you in advance and appreciate you.

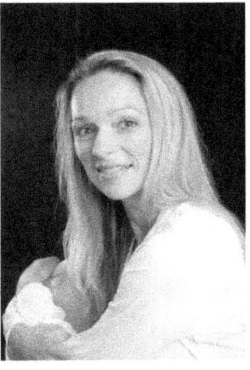

I hope that you enjoyed my book and you can check out all my other books on my website:
www.flawlesscreativewriting.com